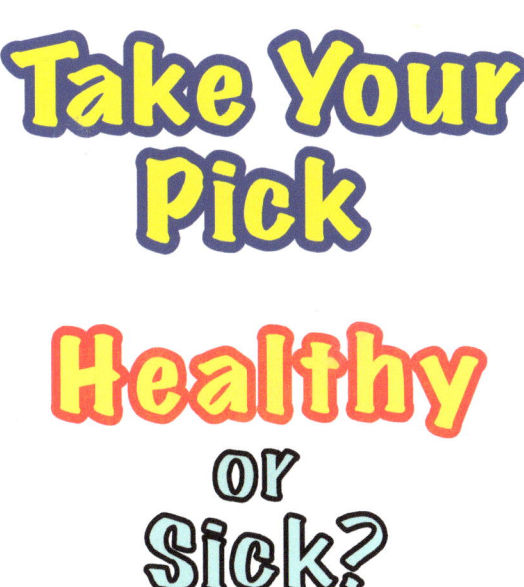

Take Your Pick

Healthy

or

Sick?

A Self-Help Guide for Kids
by Sandra Danu

Illustrations by Lisa Bohart

CreateSpace Independant Publishing Platform,
North Charleston, SC

Printed in the U.S.A. by CreateSpace,
North Charleston, SC

Take Your Pick: Healthy or Sick?
ISBN - 13: 978-1505550719
ISBN - 10: 1505550718
Library of Congress Control Number:
LCCN: 2015900251

Printed in March 2015

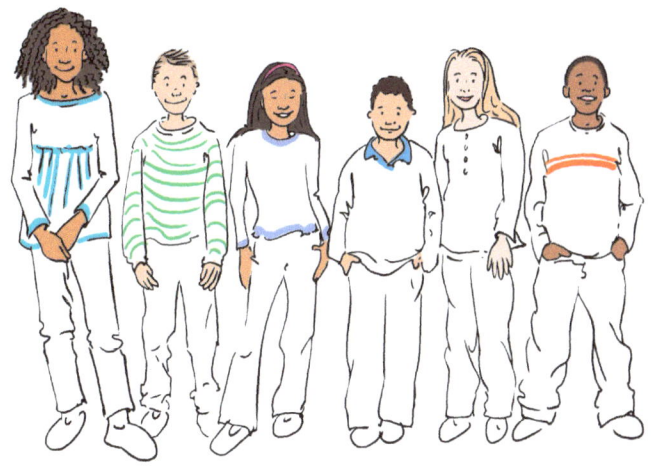

*To the next generation — may they be healthy
in body, mind, and spirit.*

Table of Contents

Introduction

I wrote this book because **a lot of kids are not as healthy as they should be**. Bad health affects bodies and brains in ways that make doing normal things much harder. Low energy, bad moods, overweight, and trouble learning are some examples. One of the main reasons for so much ill health is that people's lifestyles have changed for the worse. Lifestyle refers to what you choose to eat and do in your life as well as your attitude and your interactions with others.

Kids are the most affected by these bad habits so kids need to know what they can do to change the situation. This book will tell you how. Use it as a guide that will benefit you for the rest of your life.

Words marked with an asterisk (*) are listed in the glossary at the end of the book.

Take Your Pick: Healthy or Sick?

Healthy means that all of your parts are working the way they were designed to. When they are, you will have enough energy to do what you want to in life. Since you are a pretty complicated organism*, it can seem difficult at times to keep all of your parts performing at their best and in balance with each other. But, guess what? You don't have to figure all of that out because your body already knows how to keep you healthy. All you have to do is to give it what it needs.

Sick means that your parts are not working the way that they were designed to or that something from the outside has attacked you. It could be a germ of some kind like a virus or a bacteria or it could be a parasite* or some poisonous plant or animal. You can also become sick from bad habits. Good habits can be learned, though, and that is what this book is about. If you learn about yourself, you will see that you can be healthy your whole life... so where do we start?

First, by recognizing that you have been given great gifts that are the basis for good health— **A Body, A Mind, Emotions and Spirit!** Now you need to create good health for a lifetime by learning how to take care of them. This requires providing nourishment and protecting them from harmful influences.

At first, your parents or caregivers nourish these parts of you by providing the food your body and mind need to grow from being a baby into being a kid. They also help you to experience different emotions like love, understanding, happiness, appreciation and many other feelings. Some feelings are not pleasant like when you are angry or sad, but everyone needs to learn how to manage even the feelings we don't like. Life would be pretty boring without emotions. By asking you questions, giving you problems to solve and books to read, your parents and teachers help you to develop your mind. Your parents also help you to feel that you are part of something bigger than yourself—this whole world—and to be glad that you are not alone. This is your spiritual self.

Your Body

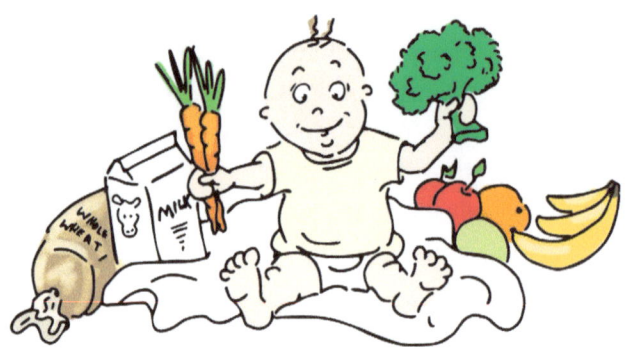

Muscles and Bones

Even though all four parts need to grow and work together, they require different "food" or material to work with. Your body has a structure that supports you. This includes your bones, muscles, tendons and ligaments and other tissues that hold you together. Muscles, which are attached to your bony skeleton, power your movement. The ones on the outside (external) allow you to use your body in many wonderful ways. How many ways can you think of that you can move thanks to these muscles? Muscles on the inside (internal) help to keep your organs like your heart, lungs and intestine working. Everything in your body has to keep moving if you are going to stay alive! Even your bones, which may look stiff and solid are always changing. The cells that make up the bones grow, die and are replaced as long as you are alive.

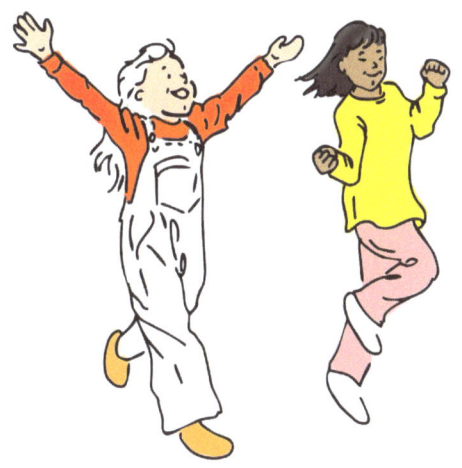

Circulation

Your body also has lots of tubes running through it to carry fluids. These tubes are called arteries, veins and capillaries. They carry your blood* to all parts of your body. Another fluid, called lymph*, gets moved around in the spaces of your body whenever your muscles move.

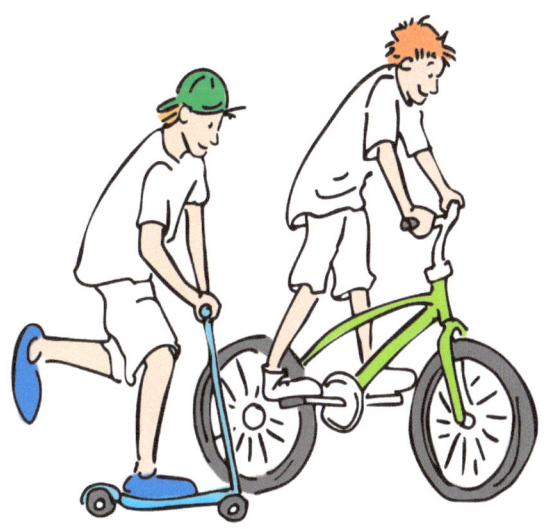

Organs

Your body includes a bunch of different organs*, each with a special job to do. There is your heart, a big muscle, that keeps your blood pumping, lungs that contract and release to keep you breathing, your stomach that partially digests your food and a 22 foot long intestine* that finishes the job. You also have special male or female organs that will make it possible for you to give life to a new human being one day—and to pass on the gift of body, mind, emotions and spirit.

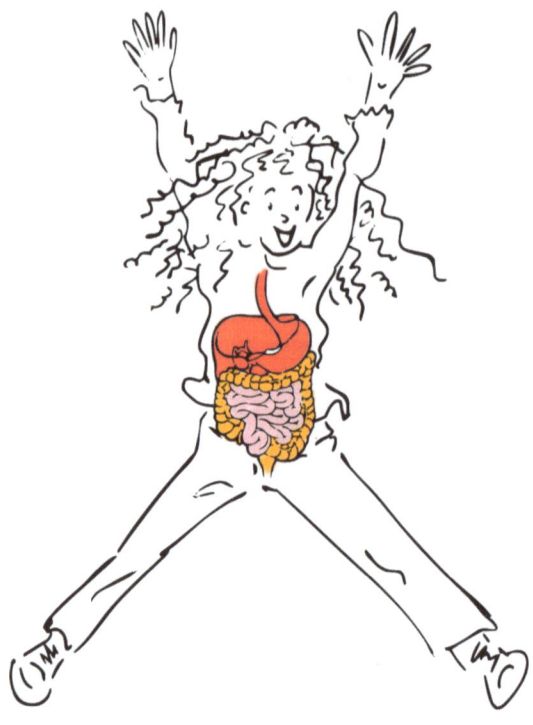

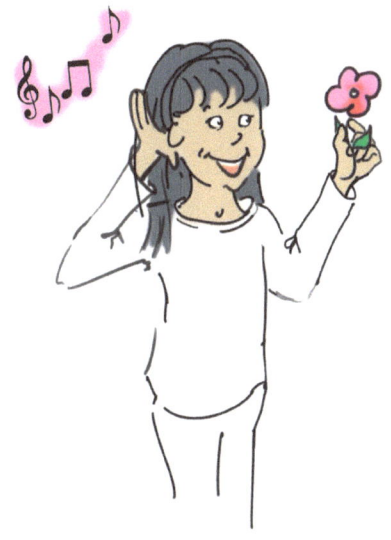

Senses

You have some organs that help you to know what is going on around you. Can you name them? Yes, eyes that see, ears that hear, a nose that smells and special parts of your mouth that make it possible for you to taste your food. There is another sense also by which you get to know the world. What is it? It is touch. There is no special location for touch—you have it all over your body. How do these senses know what to look at, listen to, smell, taste or touch? They get messages from "central command" that travel through nerves* and send messages they receive back there. What is "central command"? It is your brain.

Your Mind

The second part of the great gift you received is your mind. Your mind depends on how well your brain is working and you can do a lot to keep it working better and better throughout your life. With your mind, you can figure things out for yourself and make choices. Your mind enables you to learn—about what people in the past have known and to understand new ideas. You can even imagine things that don't exist and then create them like artists and inventors do.

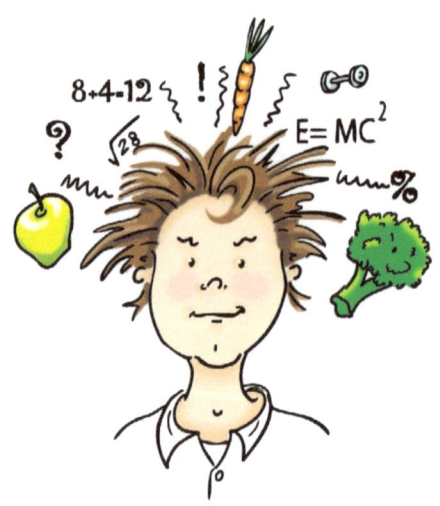

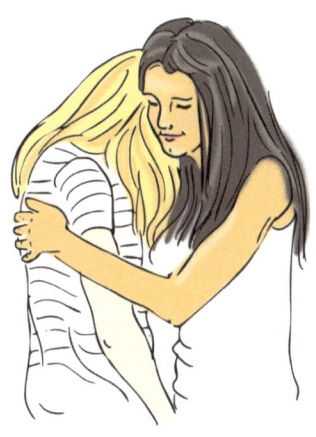

Your Emotions

Your emotions, the third gift, make it possible for you to feel something—excited to learn something about a particular subject, mad enough to take some action, grateful enough to want to thank someone. Remember that you are making the best of these gifts if they work together in a balanced way. Sometimes the emotions can be very strong and make you do something that you know, in your mind, isn't the right thing to do. It is also possible for your mind to be so busy thinking that you forget to notice your feelings. Either way, you are not balanced.

Your Spirit

Your spirit is the hardest to describe , but you know it is there. It is what makes you want to live your life in the best way possible. It has an energy that connects you to others and to the universe. If you lose your spirit, you don't want to do anything. People support their spirit in different ways, some by going to church, some by meditating, some by going out into nature. There are many ways. Whichever way you choose, it is helpful to stop your usual routine and be very quiet so that you can feel the spirit within yourself. If you listen to your spirit regularly, it will help you to make good choices in your life.

If you are very lucky, your parents made sure that you were born healthy and they continued to take care of you before you could understand what was needed. Now it is time for you to learn what it takes to stay healthy and how to take responsibility for your own health. If you do not do this, you will have problems with your body, mind, emotions, and spirit. Some problems are sickness, confusion, fear, bad relationships, lack of motivation and meaning. Problems like these mess up your life, but you can choose to prevent them—so, take your pick, healthy or sick?

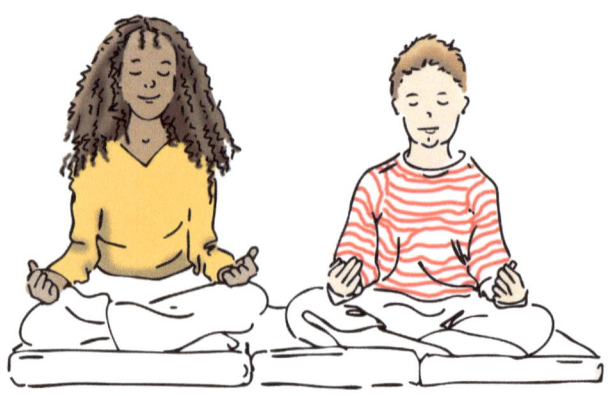

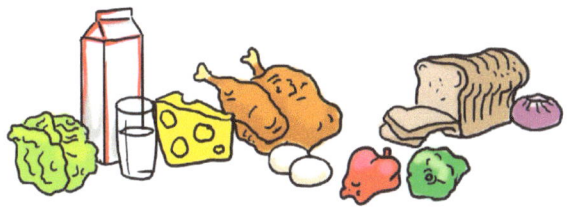

Food

What does it take to remain healthy and prevent bad things from happening in your life? First, you must feed your body, brain, emotions, and spirit with good quality food. But, you need to know the difference between poor quality and good quality food and where to get the best kind for your health. For thousands of years, when early people were exploring the world, they fished and hunted wild animals and ate wild plants and fruits. When they finally settled down in one place, they needed their food to be where they were, so they planted wild seeds and tamed animals to live on their farms. They were still eating foods that Nature had provided to make it possible for people to be strong, smart, energetic, and able to live together. Today, however, it can be harder to get the right foods for your body because the food in the supermarkets is often in packages and missing some of the things that make food healthy. These are nutrients* and include vitamins*, minerals*, enzymes*, antioxidants*, fiber, probi-otics* and more. In order to have your food work for you and not against you, you need to eat natural food that is fresh and whole.

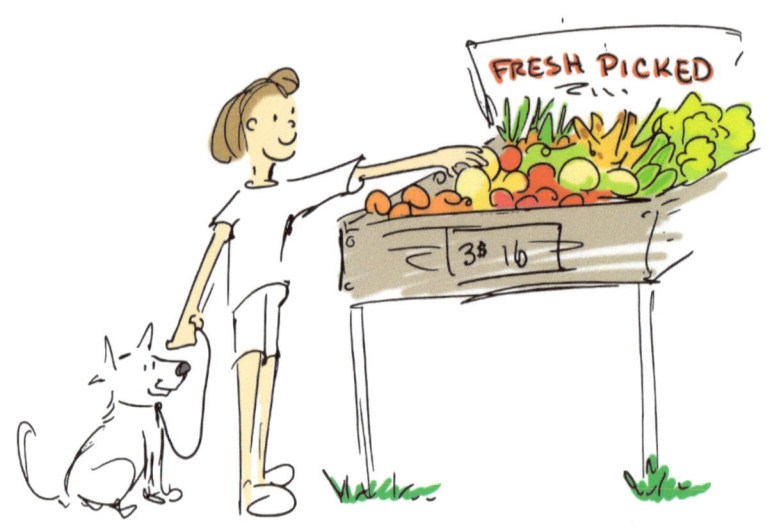

Quality* of Food

The only problem with fresh food is that it can spoil pretty quickly. Sometimes that makes farmers pick it early—before it is completely ripe. Ripe fruits and vegetables are softer and more fragile than unripe, so the farmer may pick them before they are ripe for easier transport. However, if the food is not ripe, some of the goods parts have not yet developed. Even if the green tomato gets red eventually, it doesn't taste as good and it isn't as good for you as the one that ripened on the vine. There are two clues to finding good quality food in this story. What are they? One, your sense of taste can help you tell if the food contains all of its natural elements and two, it might be better to buy food that is grown closer to home. That way it doesn't have to be picked early and will be ripe when you buy it. It is also important to buy as much organic food as you can.

Organic just means that the food is not sprayed with poisons to kill bugs or to make it grow faster. Organic food is food grown in the natural way. The seeds used to plant the crops should be natural, too, not changed by people because, like the poison sprays, they can harm you. The magic formula for quality food is natural, fresh and whole.

Natural means that it was designed by Nature, not by a company. Fresh means it is not in a package—it came from the ground or a tree not too long ago. And whole means that it has not been taken apart in some way that leaves out important parts of the original food. An example of this is flour that is used to make bread. Whole flour is made from the seeds of different kinds of grain. If you grind it up, the flour is kind of brownish. The things that are good for you in grain make it that color. White bread is bleached and the good parts of the seed are removed. This means it is not good quality food.

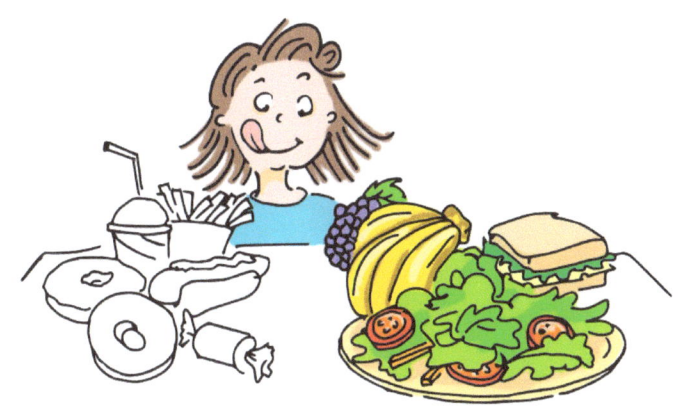

Preserving Food

Because fresh food spoils easily, people over thousands of years have figured out ways to make food last longer. Some of these methods are drying, canning*, fermenting* and freezing*, which may even keep most of the nutrients and that means that they also continue to taste good. Food prepared in all of these ways is still REAL FOOD. On the other hand, most of the preserved food we find in colorful packages in stores is more like fake food as it is mostly missing the nutrients that your body, mind, emotions, and spirit need to grow, to be strong, and to have energy. Besides lacking nutrients, those fake foods often have things added which can harm you. Some of these things are sugar, salt, artificial coloring and man-made chemicals. They may also be cooked in oil before packaging. The heat can create new compounds*, which can damage your body. Yes, sugar, salt and oil are food items and we need them, but not in the form or in the amounts they are found in 'fake food'.

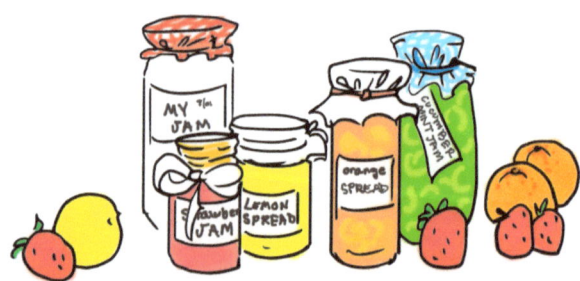

Food Groups

To make it easier to understand which kinds of foods are necessary for our health, they are divided into different food groups, each containing many foods. One of the food groups is:

Carbohydrates

This group includes sugars, starches, and grains. Carbos—the short name—give us energy and can be stored in our bodies in case we need them later. If they are in the form of a fresh potato or a whole grain, the energy is released slowly so it lasts a long time. Certain vegetables and fruits also contain carbos in a form that tastes sweet. One example is a carrot. Eating these foods is the natural way to get all of the sugar your body ever needs. Sugar provides quick energy, but it is used up quickly, too. Since pure sugar goes into your blood, this means that your blood sugar goes up and down too fast—which can make you feel sick. Refined sugar is just plain sugar, not a part of a food and is very unhealthy, even though it is used to make a lot of foods taste sweet. You probably already know that sugar can cause cavities in your teeth and make you fat, but did you know that sugar makes it harder for your body to fight off germs, uses up important nutrients like B vitamins, prevents minerals and protein from being used by your body and makes it hard for your stomach to digest food? Some people think that if you use sugar substitutes, you will avoid problems caused by sugar, but they are even worse for you. It is important to know that the only kind of sugar your body can use to make energy is glucose*. Most of the sugar added to foods and drinks to make them taste sweet is fructose*, a different form of sugar which is difficult for your body to use and ends up producing fat, not energy. Can you guess what the worst sugary, fake food is?

Soda wins! Besides having way too much sugar, it has nothing at all good in it. So, remember, to get the sugar that your brain and body needs, choose whole grain carbos that are absorbed slowly, giving you lasting energy and nutrients. If you are eating those kinds of carbos, chemicals in your brain send out a signal to stop eating when your body has as much food as it needs. So, you won't get fat from overeating. Foods that have fructose in them block that signal so you just keep on eating. Another bad form of sugar is alcohol. When someone drinks beer, wine or stronger alcoholic drinks, those drinks turn into substances that are harmful to different organs, especially the liver and the brain. Sugar and alcohol cause many of the same effects in your body that lead to diseases. Your body is designed to get rid of some alcohol and other harmful substances that you may eat, drink or breathe, but it must be healthy to do this and you cannot overload it.

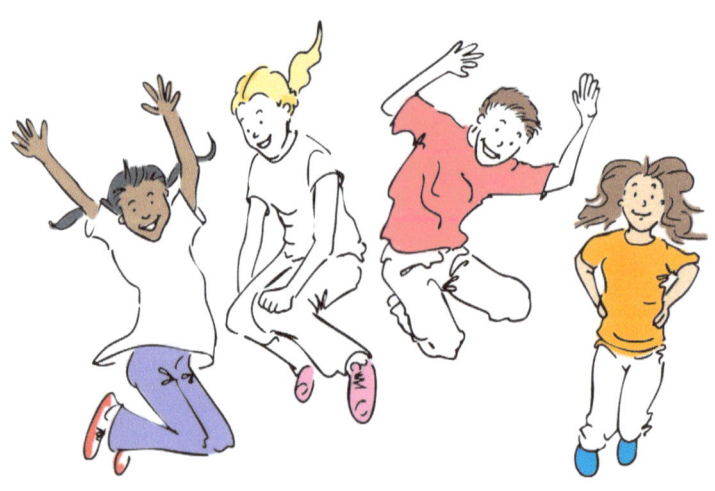

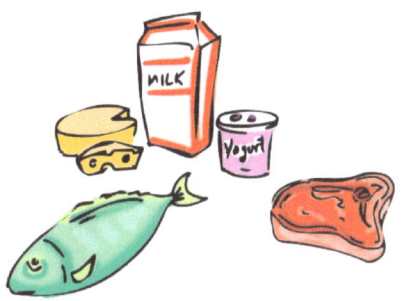

Proteins

The next food group you need is protein. Protein comes from meat and fish as well as from many plant foods like beans and nuts. You need protein to build your muscles, organs, glands, hair, nails, brain and bone. The enzymes and hormones* that control most of the functions of your body are made of proteins. Proteins form the structure of chromosomes* by which information was passed from your parents to create you. All proteins are made up of parts called amino acids*. When you eat a protein, your body breaks it down into its amino acids and then puts them back together in ways your body can use. Even though your body can make some of the proteins it needs, the rest have to be gotten from your food. These are called essential amino acids. For any one amino acid to do its job, they all have to be present. Amino acids help your brain communicate with nerve cells everywhere in your body by passing a message from one nerve to another. Vitamins and minerals, which we will discuss later, cannot work properly without them either. Also, about half of the amino acids made in your body are used to make glucose, which you now know produces energy. I think you are beginning to see that everything in your body is connected to everything else, so keeping it all in balance is the key to good health.

Fats

Fats are necessary for health, too, and like proteins, are made up of different parts or building blocks—sort of like legos where you can build many different structures using the same blocks. The building blocks of fats are called fatty acids*. For your first two years of life, you need a lot of fat to grow a normal brain. After that, you need a lot less, but enough of the right fats to maintain your nerves and cells* of all kinds as well as for back-up energy when you are not getting enough from carbos. The fats you should eat the most of are found in fatty fish, in certain vegetable oils and in nuts. You also need some of the kinds of fat found in dairy products and meat because they help your liver to make cholesterol* which is then used to make hormones. Because too much cholesterol can cause disease, you hear a lot about getting rid of it, but remember that too much or too little of anything can cause problems. The balance may be somewhat different for different people, but carbohydrates, proteins and fats are necessary for everyone.

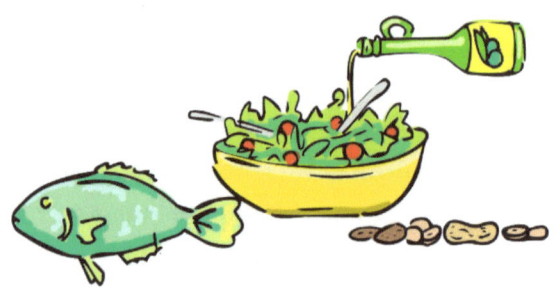

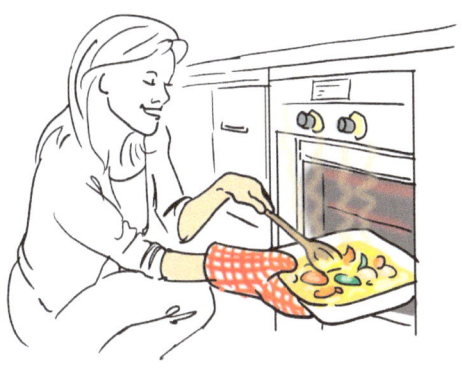

How to Treat Your Food

One of the most popular ways to prepare food is to cook it. Some ways of cooking food are healthier than others. Frying food in fat, for instance, is not healthy because the fat breaks down into harmful chemicals* when it is heated. Cooking food over a charcoal fire is not healthy if the outside gets burned because the blackened surface can harm your cells. You may think these foods taste good, but the main thing you are tasting is the fat and the salt. If you take the same food and cook it in a better way, you will taste all of the flavors of the food itself. Can you think of other ways that people cook food? Baking, boiling, and broiling are common ways to prepare food. Sometimes you need to cook it at a high temperature to kill any germs that might be in the food, but if you buy food that has been raised on healthy farms, it is usually best to cook it as little as possible. One pretty new and popular way to cook food is to use a microwave, but that method breaks the food down so you lose nutrients. Cooking this way also makes new compounds that are harmful to your body and brain. There is a lot to learn about cooking: how to keep the nutrients in the food, how to make a balanced meal and how to make it taste good.

Water

One of the most important substances to give your body is clean, fresh water. I bet you know that you can live longer without food than without water. One of the reasons for that is that you are made mostly of water. Another reason is that you need water to wash out the waste products from your body so that they don't poison you. Water is a big part of blood and lymph, fluids that carry the nutrients to all parts of your body. Water is also needed to keep minerals that you need in solution—not letting them dry up into hard deposits in your body. It is important to know what is in the water you drink. Even the chemicals that are added to water to kill germs or improve your health can sometimes be harmful. Fluoride is one of these. Bottled water may be cleaner than tap water or not, but one of the problems with it is that it usually comes in plastic bottles. Plastic can break down into little particles that get into the water and are harmful to your health. It's a good idea to ask, "what's in my water?" and "what's my water in?"

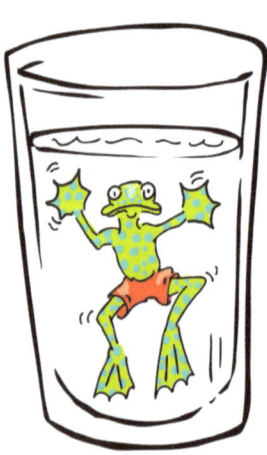

Nutrients

What exactly are these nutrients that are so important to your health? Besides the good-quality carbos, proteins and fats and good clean water, there are also micro-nutrients. "Micro" means small and we need them in very small amounts. These micro-nutrients should be present in your good-quality real food; however, sometimes there is not enough of one, or some are missing. This can happen if the plant you are eating is grown on soil that is missing some, as the plant gets its nutrients from the soil. In order to replace the missing nutrients, you may need to take some supplements.* Supplements can be vitamins, minerals, fatty acids, pro-biotics or other things your body needs. Vitamins are mostly called by letter names like A,B,C,D,E. There are many minerals that we need, too. Some of the ones you hear the most about are calcium, magnesium, potassium, sodium, iodine and iron. If you do not get everything your body needs from food and supplements, your body may not be able to build tissues, produce energy or prevent disease. Disease or sickness is the opposite of healthy and can happen to your body, mind, emotions, or spirit.

All of the measures you take to eat healthy food will benefit not only your body, but also your mind and emotions. If these parts of you do not have the nutrients they need, they can become unbalanced. If your mind is unbalanced, for instance, you may be confused, unable to think well, or imagine things are different than they really are. If your emotions are not balanced, you will overreact—become more sad, excited or frustrated than normal or you may not react enough—just not care about anything or feel like you do not have enough energy to get involved. As you can imagine, any of these situations can cause lot of problems for you and those around you. It is much easier to prevent* such problems than it is to treat them!

Exercise

Another very important part of being healthy is getting regular exercise. In order to get the most benefit from exercise, it is important to think about what kind of exercise you would enjoy. Beyond that though, you need to consider if you would be exercising your whole body—legs, arms, torso*, lungs, and heart. It must be difficult enough to cause you to work a little harder than you want to, but not so hard that you feel worn out afterwards. You should get a little out of breath and feel like your insides are exercised as well as the outside muscles. This kind of physical* exercise will stimulate* your circulation (blood and lymph we discussed), bringing oxygen* and nutrients to all parts of your body including your organs and your brain. Everything will work better as a result. Exercise also helps to balance your emotions. Your brain, emotions, and spirit need their own particular kinds of exercise to be really healthy. How do you think (oops! there's a clue) you can exercise your brain? Some ways to do it are by learning facts about any subject, training your mind to memorize a poem or story and by learning a new language. You can also practice figuring out how to solve problems or how machines work. Then, you can think about how best to use what you learn, which is an important part of being smart. For a healthy mind, you also need to be selective about the kind of information you put into your brain. You can learn to choose knowledge that is useful for a good life or you can fill your mind with harmful ideas and thoughts. If you have a healthy mind, you will be able to make good decisions for yourself. If not, you could be influenced too much by others and not be able to judge whether something is a good idea or not. Your brain can continue to grow for your whole life if it is healthy.

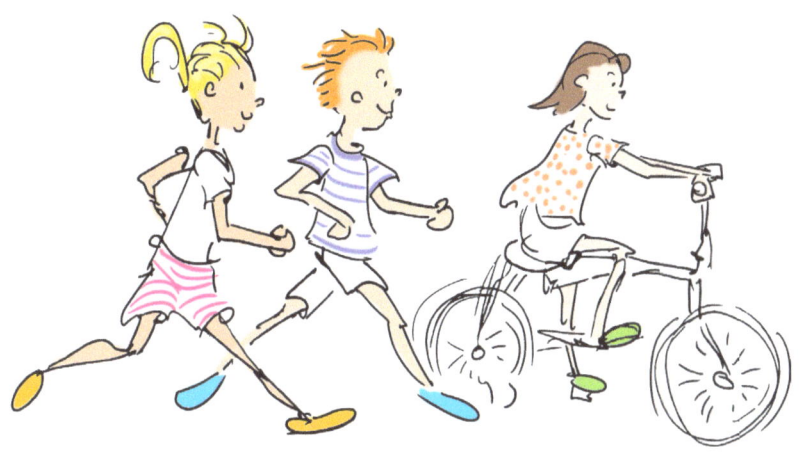

Exercising emotions may seem a little strange, but if you think of exercising as "using" and "keeping in good shape", it is not so strange. The first step is to observe how you feel, what makes you feel that way and how you react when someone else makes you feel a certain way. In other words, you need to learn a lot about how you are expressing your feelings and how that is affecting your health and the relationships you have with other people. After that, you can try to express your emotions in a way that may get better results than if you are not even noticing. Better results means that both you and the people you are with feel good about your interactions.

All of these suggestions for exercise require work. Without the work you don't get strong and able to deal with challenges and problems whether they are with your body, mind, emotions, or spirit. So remember—health is not ever about only one thing—everything needs to be in balance.

To help you achieve that balance or see more clearly what is missing, spiritual exercises are helpful. Start by finding some-place quiet and sit with a straight spine. Cross-legged on the floor is a good choice. Now, just try to notice your body, your mind and your emotions without changing them. If you do not inter-fere, they will all calm down by themselves. If you do this often enough, you will strengthen your spirit.

What to Know About Physical Exercise

- *Do it Daily:* Needed to keep your parts working well
- *Warm Up:* Cold muscles and joints cause injuries
- *Vary It:* Do stretches, runs and jumps
- *Work Hard:* Pushing your body a little makes it stronger; too much causes stress
- *Cool Down:* Slow down gradually, then relax muscles
- *Tip:* Remember to drink water before and after; when it's hot, you might need to add minerals

Elimination

Now, eating right and exercising should prevent any kind of illness because such a program feeds and tones your body and helps it to eliminate* waste products and toxins*. Elimination is very important for your health! Your body will naturally get rid of some waste material, by deep breathing, sweating, peeing (urinating), and other mechanisms, but the most important is pooping. A lot of people don't like talking about pooping, so problems are often ignored. Pooping is essential to get rid of waste products—stuff left over after your body has used what it needs from your food. If you do not poop at least once a day, the waste left in your body will poison your body, mind, emotions, and spirit. Your body gets used to a regular routine, so it is best to pick a time of day to poop that is the same every day. Just after a breakfast of fruit and whole grains (which help your intestine to work) is a good time. Move around a little, then relax on the toilet. If you have to get up a little earlier than usual to have time for this, do it. It will be worth it as you will feel your best all day long. If you are doing the right things to be healthy and still don't poop easily and regularly, you may not have enough acid in your stomach or probiotics in your intestine. These can easily be supplemented and a naturopath* or a nutritionist* can tell you how much to take.

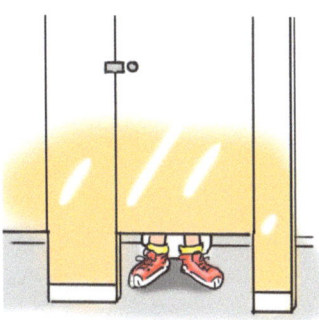

What Else?

There is something else that you need in order to be healthy. Can you guess what it is? You can't see it, touch it, taste it, hear it or smell it, but it is real and very important. It is sleep—you need a good 8 hours of sleep a night because your body, mind, emotions, and spirit need time to recover from all of the work they do all day long. All of your parts rest and rebuild during sleep. Your body is designed to respond to light and darkness so it is best to go to sleep about when it is getting dark and wake up when it is getting light outside. You do not have to be exact, but understand that you function best if you stick fairly closely to that guideline. Other things can tell you when you need to sleep, too. If you are tired during the day, you are probably not getting enough sleep at night. Babies and teenagers actually need a lot of sleep as they are both growing very fast. If you have been very active physically or mentally during the day or had a rough day emotionally, you will need more sleep to recover. Remember though, that first you need to get in balance. Otherwise, you may not have a restful sleep. You do this through activities that are different from those that caused the fatigue. If you studied too hard, you should exercise your body a little before trying to sleep; if you ran too hard, read an interesting book in a relaxed position. Can you think of other ways to get back in balance? It is not a good idea to watch TV, to use your phone or computer or to be in artificial bright light before bed. Those things are too stimulating and so make it harder to become calm and in balance, which is necessary for healthy sleep. If you feel sleepy, go to bed. Fighting off sleep can make it harder to fall asleep when you want to.

Making Good Choices

Sometimes it is quite tricky to make good decisions about your health. Very often, when something new is invented or created, it seems like the best thing in the world. Later people realize, that the wonderful thing also has some problems. One example is electronics*. All of the new phones, computers, televisions, computers, and other gadgets may make life easier or more fun, but they also mean you can never get away from the continual messages. This creates stress*, and stress is not healthy. To get back in balance, you need to take a break from all of that and do something entirely different. Another problem is that being close to anything electronic like a cell phone held to your ear, or sitting too near the TV or using a hair dryer can mean that these electronic appliances are affecting the electricity in your body—probably not in a good way. The atoms* in your body carry an electric charge and messages move along your nerves by electric charge—these can be affected by an outside source of electricity. Something else that people developed and thought was a big improvement are medicines that are used to kill bugs or germs. Then people learned that you need a balance of good bugs and germs in your body and they get killed off with the bad ones. Chemicals used to grow food can also get transferred to your body. Solutions to problems are not always easy. Being able to consider all sides of a problem is part of having a healthy brain and will help you to come up with the best solution. So, there are two general actions needed for good health. One is to choose the things that are good for you like good food and experiences that help you to grow. The other is NOT to choose things that are bad for you.

Sometimes, not choosing means to just get away—get away from the junk food isle in the market, get away from the poisons that are sprayed near you, get away from any message that is ugly, mean or violent to you or someone else. Remember that there are always choices. It is up to you to choose what is best for you. If you are actively involved in your own life, instead of just letting things happen, those who are trying to get you to make bad choices will fail. Try to think of different kinds of situations where you would have to make a choice and how you would decide what the best choice is.

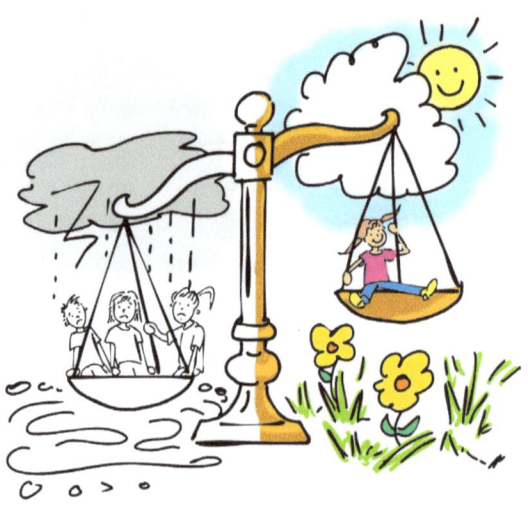

Take Action

Now that you know what is required for good health, how do you—as a kid—make sure that you are healthy? The best way is to let your parents or caregivers know that you would really appreciate it if they will help you. You can ask them to provide fresh food that is not contaminated* with pesticides*, hormones or germs. You can offer to help shop so that a variety of vegetables and fruits as well as nuts, seeds, eggs and other foods providing important nutrients will be available in your home. You can suggest that no unhealthy food be bought. If they choose to eat unhealthy foods themselves, you can still request that they buy good food for you. You can also ask for opportunities to do activities outside of school that exercise your body, brain, and emotions. There are all kinds of sports, many interesting questions in life to investigate through clubs or activities, and many expressive arts to experience. Though it is healthy to have interests and be able to pursue them by yourself, it is also important to engage with others who may have the same interests. Many times you can find such groups or teams in the school setting. Sometimes you have to look around your city or town to see what is available. If you can't find it, you could start a club yourself. It is also important to try something new once in a while.

Even though your parents or caregivers may help you to be healthy, you will have to take more and more responsibility yourself as you get older. You can do this by making smart choices. This takes having a lot of information so you need to continue to educate yourself. Look around at people who don't seem well and try to understand what wrong choices they might have made.

There are many reasons why it can be hard to make smart choices. One is the fact that your environment, the world around you, contains a lot of chemicals that can be harmful to your health. These can be found in the soil in which your food is grown, in the water you drink and in the air you breathe. A lot of these chemicals are used because they are helpful for farming, as medicines, to kill germs, or for other good reasons, but there are now so many of them that they are also causing a lot of health problems.

People have to learn how to reduce their exposure. For instance, there are ways to keep bugs out of your house without poisoning them and yourself. And, as we said before, you can choose to eat organic food instead of food that has been grown with poisons.

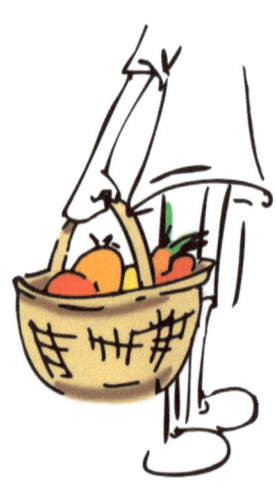

Another difficult choice could be when people tell you that you don't need to work at solving your problems. They may say that all you need to do is to take something to forget about them. Drugs* are everywhere today, but people who offer them to you never admit that they have very bad effects after they make you feel good for a short while. Drugs will change the way your mind and emotions work, so you could feel happy when you were just sad or feel like everything is going real well even when it is not. Drugs seem to change reality, but they don't. They just change your brain. These brain changes also make you feel like you have to have the drugs. This means you are no longer able to make healthy choices. The need to have drugs is called addiction*. You can also be addicted to other things besides drugs. They are an example of something you put into your body, but you can get addicted to certain kinds of activities, too, that get you badly out of balance. The one thing that all addictions have in common is that they are a way to avoid facing real life.

Allowing yourself to become addicted is one of the worst ways to waste the gifts that we have been given. If you are healthy, you understand that everyone has problems, bad days and even failures, but you also know that you can just take a break, do something to take your mind off of it and go back later to solve the problem. A healthy person does not destroy himself or herself because life is not always perfect. A healthy person even thinks that "perfect" can be boring and it's good to have a problem to solve to keep things interesting!

What else might make it hard for you to have a healthy life? Can you figure out how to deal with that?

Sickness

We discussed how poor health habits can cause bad moods, make you feel sad a lot of the time, not be able to think clearly or have the strength to do the things you want to do. Those effects should be a warning to you—if you don't apply what you know about being healthy, you may get a disease*. People can become sick very quickly if they get a germ or infection* or if some part of their body is damaged, but most disease is the result of not living a healthy lifestyle over a fairly long time. You need to pay attention to the signs that your body, mind, or emotions are not working as well as they should be before the situation turns into a disease. At that point, it is much more difficult to get healthy again. I hope you now see that you don't have to be afraid that you will get sick—you know how to choose to stay healthy. I think I know how you will answer the challenge of this book: "Take your pick—healthy or sick?"

**Signs that you are *not* healthy —
better get with the program!**

- Low energy; tired a lot of the time
- Feeling sick to your stomach
- Being overweight or too skinny
- Not pooping often enough
- Feeling weak; looking pale
- Having cold hands and feet
- Having a cough, a rash or a sore throat
- Hurting in different parts (body, mind, emotions, spirit)
- Other bad feelings that won't go away

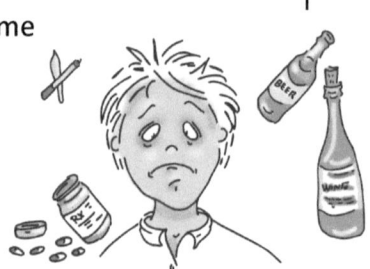

Prevention

Very many health problems can be prevented if you develop a healthy lifestyle as I have described. Even if a bad germ comes along, your body will be better able to fight it because your immune system* will be strong. Because we cannot control everything in our environment, you may need expert help to improve a health situation that seems out of balance. If it has to do with allergies, asthma, ear infections, bad reactions to foods, stomach problems and many other general conditions, you can get help from a naturopath or a nutritionist. If you have some particular weakness like bad eyesight, you need to go to an eye doctor. For a sudden serious disease or because you've been hurt, you may need to go to another kind of medical doctor or even to a hospital. Just remember that medicine means drugs. As we learned earlier, drugs can do you harm even if they sometimes are necessary. The best idea is to avoid them as much as possible by working on being healthy.

Remember

Eat well and feel swell
Lazy is wrong if you want to be strong
Feeling bad, or glad or sad?
It's quite alright to sigh or cry
And when you know you need a lift
Trust in the power of each great gift!

Glossary

Some words can be used in different ways; the following definitions are how they are used in this book.

Addiction— a powerful and harmful need to take something into your body or to do something

Amino Acid— one of several acids containing nitrogen which make up a main part of proteins

Antioxidant— a substance that reduces damage done by oxygen

Atom— the smallest possible unit of a chemical element and the basis for all matter in the universe

Blood— red fluid carrying oxygen and nutrients through our arteries and veins

Canning— a method of preserving food in glass jars or cans

Cell— a tiny unit of plant or animal life which has a nucleus (center) surrounded by a membrane

Chemicals— elements that make up matter and give it a certain character

Cholesterol— a fatty element necessary for life; found in cells and body fluids

Chromosome— The part of a cell that contains the genes which control how an animal or a plant grows and what it becomes.

Compound— a substance made up of two or more elements

Contaminate— make impure by contacts or mixing

Disease— a condition that causes harm to a person internally

Drug— a substance that causes chemical changes in the body

Electronics— study of the movement of free electrons (particles with a negative charge)

Eliminate— to get rid of

Enzyme— a protein that helps a chemical reaction take place within a living organism

Fatty Acids— a specific type of acid found in certain foods

Fermentation— a change brought about by yeast

Freezing— making cold enough to harden and preserve

Fructose— a sugar that occurs naturally in fruits and honey

Glucose— a type of sugar found in plants

Hormones— a substance produced in the body that influences how it grows and develops

Immune system— a network of cells, tissues, and organs that work together to protect the body against infection

Infection— the invasion and multiplication of micro-organisms e.g. viruses, bacteria and parasites that do not normally live in the body

Intestine— same as the bowel; the tube that runs from the stomach to the anus where food is processed, absorbed, and eventually eliminated.

Lymph— an almost colorless fluid that travels through its own system of vessels; it contains cells that help fight infection and disease

Mineral— a substance that is formed in the earth and is not a plant or animal

Naturopath— a person who has received an advanced degree to teach how to be healthy

Nerves— fibers coming out of the spine and connecting to all parts of the body; messages move along these fibers to tell different parts what to do

Nutrient— a plant or animal element which benefits our bodies when eaten

Nutritionist— a person who studies food and its nutrients

Organ— a group of body tissues organized into a particular structure to serve a specific function

Organism— a living individual made up of several organs and other parts that work together to maintain life and health.

Oxygen— an element found in water, air, rocks and minerals that can combine with most other elements; it is essential for life

Parasite— an animal or plant that lives in or on another animal or plant and gets food and/or protection from it

Pesticide— a chemical for destroying unwanted bugs

Physical— having to do with the body

Prevention— keeping something from happening

Probiotics— germs that are necessary for good health

Quality— a grade of excellence

Stimulate— to bring about activity or action

Stress— physical, mental, or emotional tension or that which causes it

Supplement— a nutrient or other substance added to one's diet

Torso— the part of the body between the base of the neck and the top of the legs

Toxin— poison

Vitamin— a substance needed for normal health and functioning of the body; we get them through food or supplements.

www.ingramcontent.com/pod-product-compliance
Lightning Source LLC
Chambersburg PA
CBHW050847290526
45792CB00002B/551